Mental Status
Core Skills Guid   ve

Text Copyright 2(
Nick Fitzgerald, I   _ . ..zgerald, R.N

Table of Contents

Introduction

Welcome to this comprehensive core skills guide relating to the mental status examination (MSE). The guide will lead you through the MSE in a structured and systematic manner, providing examples and prompt questions of each key element, as your learning progresses.

Chapter 1: Specific Learning Objectives

Describe the mental status examination and the 9 key elements and provide examples.

Describe the qualities of the assessor and provide examples.

Describe how each of the 9 key elements of the mental status examination relate to an individuals mental health status and provide examples.

Describe a variety of assessment terminology and explain how the terminology can be integrated into each assessment.

Chapter 2: What is the mental status examination?

The mental status examination (MSE) is a methodical assessment tool used to evaluate the appearance, behaviour, and general manner and functioning of an individual. Karl Jaspers, a German – Swiss psychiatrist and philosopher, has been attributed with pioneering the MSE in 1912, as a structure to develop his ideas to obtain both systematic and person-centered evidence to understand human behaviour.

The MSE provides an accurate picture of an individual's mental health status, at any moment in time, and is considered to be a significant factor in the comprehensive assessment process.

Clinicians naturally assess elements of the MSE when they perform their daily observations and tasks. The data collected from an MSE is invaluable in assessing the individual's ability to function. The findings of the MSE will also identify if further mental health follow-up and interventions are required. Mental health rating scales, such as the Hamilton Rating Scale for Anxiety or the Patient Health Questionnaire (PHQ-9) can also be used in the assessment of an individual's mental health status that can inform risk assessment and risk management planning.

Chapter 3: What qualities should the assessor possess?

There are many qualities and skills that the assessor should possess, in order to develop an appropriate therapeutic relationship and engage individuals in the assessment and treatment process.

These include:

The ability to build rapport so that confidence and trust can be established.

The ability to be non-judgmental so that the assessor is not disapproving of others choices, even when they do not agree with the individual's or others choices.

The ability to be empathic so that the assessor is in tune with the individual's thoughts and feelings.

The ability to actively listen so that the assessor can improve their understanding and give their full attention using verbal and non-verbal communication skills to what is being reported. Tone of voice, facial expression, body language and brief verbal responses can all be used to reinforce to the individual that the assessor is being fully attentive.

The ability to be systematic so that all the data is obtained, in order to make informed decisions.

The ability to be objective so that the assessor is not influenced by their own or others personal feelings and makes informed decisions based on the evidence.

The ability to be observant so that the assessor is attentive and aware of any changes in the individual's presentation or message that they are reporting.

Chapter 4: What are the 9 key elements of the mental status examination?

Appearance.

Behaviour.

Speech.

Mood and Affect.

Form of Thought.

Content of Thought.

Perception.

Orientation and Sensorium.

Insight and Judgement.

Chapter 5: Appearance

Assessing an individual's appearance through observation can provide clues to their level of functioning. The assessor should consider the social context in which the individual's appearance is being observed and assessed. Assessing an individual's appearance in isolation of behavioural or other factors will not provide an objective assessment of their mental health status.

For example, an individual who is wearing flamboyant or bizarre clothing, a lot of jewellery and make-up, alongside their observed behaviour, pattern of speech, and form and content of thought, may be indicative that they may or may not be experiencing a manic-type episode. An individual who is wearing dirty clothing may be indicative that they are experiencing psychosis, depression, they are homeless or they do not have access to a washing machine.

It is imperative that the assessor accurately describes the individual's appearance, which will include their apparent age, height, weight and grooming. An individual who appears older than their apparent age might be suggestive of self-neglect, ill health, malnutrition or other lifestyle factors.

For example, recent significant weight loss may be indicative of physical ill health, substance misuse, low mood, eating problems or manic or anxiety-related issues, or they cannot afford to buy food. Asking further questions relating to issues, such as weight loss or their health issues will add further evidence to the assessment. A description of their appearance may also include hairstyle, tattoos, facial hair, scars and piercings. This list is not exhaustive and the assessor should provide as much detail as possible.

Prompt questions
Do they appear to be younger or older than their apparent age?

Is their build tall, short, thin or obese? Provide weight and height if possible.

Is their clothing appropriate to their age, season, setting and occasion?

Is their clothing clean, neat, tidy, precise or threadbare?

Is their make up applied correctly, cautiously or negligently?

Does their hygiene and grooming appear clean, precise or do they appear unwashed and grubby?

Does their hair appear well groomed or dirty?

Does their odour smell of sweat, deodorant, alcohol or other odour?

Do they have a beard or moustache?

Do they have tattoos or scars? Provide detail.

Are they wearing jewellery? Provide detail.[1]

Appearance example

David Smith is a 42-year old Australian male. David reports that he is 185 cm tall and weighs 90 kilograms, and he appears to be of normal build. David appears younger than his stated age and he is wearing clean clothing that consists of a short-sleeved t-shirt, shorts, running shoes, a baseball cap and sunglasses, which are appropriate for the weather, as it is warm and sunny at the time of the assessment. David's hygiene appears intact and he has short clean and well-groomed hair and there is no evidence of body odour. David reports that he had a shower prior to the assessment.

Chapter 6: Behaviour

Behaviour can be expressed as both verbal and non-verbal and can be used to identify an individual's emotional and mental state. Behaviour may include body language, psychomotor agitation, gestures, posture, gait, eye contact, response to the assessment itself, and rapport and social engagement.[2]

Prompt questions

Does their facial expression appear sad, confused, nervous, frightened, sullen, absent-minded, uninterested, vacant, shocked, stressed or cheerful, reactive, engrossed, energetic, excited or thrilled?

Do they appear kind, interactive, attentive or oppositional, muddled or disinterested?

Does their eye contact appear indirect, unchanging, passing, obvious, fleeting or no eye contact given?

Is their way of walking and pace slow, cautious, trundling, normal, hurried, thrusting, staggering or awkward?

Is their handshake firm, warm to touch, cool to touch, strong, delicate, light, drawn out, declined or over familiar?

Do they display unusual movements, such as grimaces, tics, twitches, spasms, foot tapping, handwringing, repetitive behaviour, mannerisms, posturing, nail biting, or pointless duplication and replication of others movement?

Is their posture deformed, rigid, unsteady, slumped, upright, exhibiting odd characteristics, bending down or comfortable?

Is their speed of movement restless, measured, deliberate, delayed or disturbed?

Is their co-ordination uncoordinated, uncomfortable, alert or reactive?

Do they display anger, dissatisfaction, confrontation, antagonism, despondency or pleasure?

Are they participating in the MSE or do they seem disconnected, bored or intense?

Behaviour example

David's facial expression appears sad, as evidenced by his continued tearfulness and he reports that his dog passed away today. David appears kind and interactive, as he is able to engage in conversation appropriately with obvious eye contact throughout the assessment. David does not appear uncoordinated and his rate of movement appears normal. David appears to actively engage in the assessment and he does not display any agitation, confrontation or dissatisfaction. David states *"thank you for listening to me"*.

Chapter 7: Speech

The assessment of an individual's speech can identify if they are experiencing a variety of mental disorders. For example, an individual who presents in a fast, rambling and loud manner that is out of character for them may be experiencing a manic-type episode. An individual presenting with slow, hesitant, mumbling and monotonous speech may be experiencing low mood, which may result in them finding it difficult to express themselves adequately. However, it is important to note that a variety of speech patterns may also relate to other disorders, so it is imperative that the assessor completes a descriptive account of the individual's speech pattern and note any changes from the norm.

Prompt questions

Is their rate of speech fast, slow or normal?

Is their flow of speech normal, cautious, long-winded, faltering, extroverted, stuttering, erratic, exhibiting long pauses or absent mindedness?

Is their speech volume loud, normal, shouting, gentle, quiet or indistinct?

Is their speech clear, indistinct, inarticulate, long-winded, applicable or disjointed?

Does their speech display energy, boredom, monotony, normalcy, force, stress or unpredictability?

Is their quality of speech responsive only to questions, offers information, limited, silent, expressed in more words that needed or repetitive?

Speech example

David's speech appears to be of normal rate, flow and volume. David does not appear to raise his voice during the course of the interview. He appears coherent and his responses appear relevant to the conversation. David displays normal responsiveness to the assessor questions and he appears to offer normal quantity of information.

Chapter 8: Mood and Affect

Assessing an individual's mood and affect are important elements of the MSE. Affect refers to the assessor's objective description of the individual's facial expressions of emotion. Mood refers to the individual's subjective description of their emotional experiences.

The individual describes their internal feelings or emotions that often influence their behaviour and their perception of the world, and is their subjective description and opinion of their internal feelings. For example, the individual might describe their mood as *happy* or *sad*. Affect describes the individual's objective external emotional response, which is observed by the assessor. For example, the assessor might objectively describe the individual's affect as *normal*, *restricted*, *blunted* or *flat*.

- Normal affect relates to changes in an individual's facial and vocal expressions and the use of their body language.
- Restricted affect relates to the depletion in the individual's range of expression and effort.
- Blunted affect relates to the drastic depletion of the individual's range of affect.
- Flat affect relates to the absence in the individual's affect. For example, their

communication may be monotone and their facial features unmoving.

The assessor will also determine if the individual's mood and affect are congruent (consistent) or incongruent (inconsistent). For example, if the individual's affect is observed and described by the assessor as *flat*, but the individual describes their mood as *happy*, their mood and affect will be incongruent (inconsistent) and further clarification will be required. Also, if the individual describes their mood as *depressed*, and their affect is observed and described as *blunted* by the assessor, it can be determined that their mood and affect are congruent.

Other words and definitions that assessors often use include:
- Euphoric - elevated or exceedingly happy.
- Euthymic - even mood, with normal ups and downs.
- Dysthymic - depressed for more than 2 years.
- Irritable - easily annoyed and provoked to anger.
- Labile - easily altered and liable to change.
- Fearful - feeling or showing fear or anxiety.

- Hostile - feeling or showing opposition or dislike.[1]

Prompt questions
How do they describe their mood?
How would you accurately describe their affect?
Is their mood and affect congruent or incongruent?

Mood and Affect example
David describes his mood, as *"I'm not feeling too happy at the moment as my dog passed away today and I feel really sad"*. David's affect appears flat, which is appropriate to the situation he describes. David appears tearful throughout the interview. David's mood and affect appear congruent.

Chapter 9: Form of Thought

Form of thought is characterized by the structure and understanding of thoughts that are articulated through an individual's speech or expression of ideas. Form of thought can be described as logical, illogical, relevant or irrelevant to the subject matter.

Other words and definitions assessors often use include:

- Unrelated comments such as *loose associations* or *derailment*.
- Regular changes of subject such as *flight of ideas* or *tangential thinking*.
- Unrestricted ambiguity such as *circumstantial thinking*.
- Gibberish words such as *word salad*.
- Forced or stopped speech such as *thought racing* or *blocking*.

Form of Thought signs and symptoms

Circumstantial thinking: Slowed thinking incorporating unnecessary trivial details. Eventually the goal of the thought is reached.

Clang associations: Speech in which words are chosen because of their sounds rather than their meanings.

Confabulation: A plausible but imagined memory that fills in gaps in what is remembered.

Derailment: A pattern of speech in which an individual's ideas slip off one track onto another that is completely unrelated.

Echolalia: The repetition or echoing of verbal utterances made by another person.

Flight of ideas: Speech consists of a stream of accelerated thoughts with abrupt changes from topic to topic and no central direction.

Loose associations: Speech characterized by slipping from one train of thought to another loosely related train of thought.

Mutism: A refusal to speak.

Neologisms: The use of a newly made up word, or an everyday word used in an idiosyncratic way.

Overvalued idea: An unreasonable and sustained belief that is maintained with less than delusional intensity.

Perseveration: Mental operations carry on past the point that they serve as a function. For example, *"What day is it?" "Monday". "What time is it?" "Monday"*.

Poverty of speech: Less speech than normal.

Tangentiality: Replying to a question in an oblique or irrelevant way.

Thought blocking: Repeated and abrupt halt to speech as a result of losing ones train of thought.

Word salad: Speech that is an incoherent and incomprehensible mix of words and phrases.[2]

Prompt questions

Would you describe their form of thought as logical, illogical, relevant or irrelevant to the subject matter?

Are they regularly changing the subject matter?

Are they making irrelevant comments and going off track from the subject matter?

Are they talking gibberish or word salad?

What other assessment terminology can you use to describe their form of thought?

Form of Thought example

David's thought form appears logical and relevant to the conversation. David responds to each question logically and does not appear to offer illogical responses. For example, David was asked, "*Tell me more about your dog*". David's response was "*my dog was a Border collie and his name was Duke. I know that he passed away today and I miss him terribly*". David's response appears relevant to the subject matter. David does not appear to display any abnormal form of thought.

Chapter 10: Content of Thought

An individual's thinking can be appraised according to their thought content, which can be described as the experience of delusions, overvalued ideas, preoccupations, depressive thoughts, obsessions, anxiety and self-harm, aggression, and suicidal and homicidal ideation.

The assessor will explore the individual's thought content with additional questioning to elicit understanding with regard to intensity and salience, the extent to which the thoughts are experienced as their own and under their control and the degree of belief or conviction associated with the thoughts.[3]

Delusions

A delusion can be defined as a false fixed belief, which is out of keeping with the individual's educational, cultural and social background and is held with extraordinary conviction and subjective certainty. Delusions are described as persecutory, grandiose, referential, erotomanic, jealous and misidentified.[4]

The definition of each delusion type:

• Persecutory delusion: The conviction that harm will arise or is going to arise.

• Grandiose delusion: The conviction that the individual possesses greater authority or powers.

- Referential delusion: The conviction that external proceedings or objects have particular meaning to them.
- Erotomanic delusion: The conviction that another individual is in love or adores them.
- Jealous delusion: The conviction that a spouse or significant other is being adulterous (Othello syndrome).
- Misidentified delusion: The conviction that a spouse or close relative has been replaced by an identical-looking pretender (Capgras delusion).
- Thought broadcast: The conviction that an individual's thoughts are being transmitted out loud so that others can hear them.
- Thought insertion: The conviction that an individual's thoughts are not their own, but are in their mind.
- Thought withdrawal: The conviction that an individual's thoughts are being taken out by another indiviual.[5]

Content of Thought signs and symptoms
Overvalued ideas: A false and sustained conviction that is held but not with delusional intensity. For example, an individual with a belief that they are the greatest cricketer in the world but have never played cricket.[5]

Obsessions: A repeated and constant thought, urge or image that is unwanted, troublesome and invasive thought that cannot be repressed by the individual.[5]

Phobias: An intense irrational dread of or aversion to something.

Pre-occupations:
Thoughts that are not rigid, untrue or disturbing but have undue importance in the individual's mind. Preoccupations that can be clinically significant include thoughts of suicide, homicide, suspiciousness or fearful convictions. The assessment of suicidal or homicidal risk includes detailed questions about the nature of the individual's suicidal or homicidal thoughts, beliefs about death, reasons for living and whether they have made any specific plans to end their own life or another individual's life.

Prompt questions
Do they appear intense and emotional?
Do they appear in control of their thoughts?
Are their thoughts unusual and are they fixed?
Are they expressing delusional beliefs and what type are they?
Is there any other evidence of thought disorder?

Content of Thought example

David does not appear to be experiencing, nor does he admit to, any current delusions, over-valued ideas, obsessions, phobias, preoccupations and harmful thoughts towards himself or others. David does not express any risk concerns relating to his own health or the health of others. David expresses his current preoccupation with the death of his dog, however it is not clinically significant and it is in context with his current experience of grief and loss. David states that, *"if I need extra support regarding the death of Duke I will get it, but my family and friends have said that they will support me to organize a funeral and celebration for my dog in the next few days"*.

Chapter 11: Perception

A perception is any sensory experience, such as hallucinations, pseudo - hallucinations and illusions.

Hallucinations

Hallucinations are defined as an apparent perception that is not present. There are 5 types of hallucinations that occur in the 5 senses. They include auditory (hearing), visual (seeing), tactile (touch), olfactory (smell) and gustatory (taste) hallucinations.

• Auditory hallucinations include second-person hallucinations that talk to the individual that can be threatening and insulting, and third person hallucinations that talk about the individual and are thoughts heard by them spoken aloud. Command hallucinations instruct the individual to undertake a particular action, which may have significant negative consequences to the individual being commanded.

• Visual hallucinations involve sight that can consist of formed images such as other individuals.

• A pseudo-hallucination is an externalized sensory image vivid enough to be a hallucination but recognized as unreal.[6]

An illusion is defined as a false idea or belief that the individual accepts as not being real.

Prompt questions
Is there any evidence, either overt or hidden, that suggests they are experiencing any form of hallucination?
Is there any evidence, either overt or hidden, that suggests they are experiencing any form of delusion?
Is there any evidence, either overt or hidden, that suggests they are experiencing any form of illusion?
Is there any evidence of risk to themselves or others?

Perception example
David does not appear to be experiencing any current perceptual disturbance, as evidenced by his current denial of suffering from hallucinations, delusions or illusions. David denies any history of experiencing perceptual disturbance.

Chapter 12: Orientation and Sensorium

Orientation and sensorium refers to an individual's current capacity to process information.

The assessment terminology that assessor's use to assess and obtain data relating to an individual's orientation and sensorium include:

• Level of consciousness - alert, drowsy, intoxicated or stuporous (not quite fully conscious).

• Orientation to reality - expressed in regard to time, place and person.

• Memory function - relates to both short-term and long-term memory.

• Literacy and mathematics skills.

• Visuo-spatial processing - copying a diagram or drawing a bicycle.

• Attention and concentration - observations about the level of distractibility or performance on a mentally challenging task.

• General knowledge.

• Language - naming objects and following instructions.

• Ability to deal with abstract concepts - existing in thought, or as an idea but not having a physical or concrete existence, such as love.

Prompt questions
What is their level of consciousness?
Are they orientated to time, place and person?
Are they able to recall short-term and long-term events?
Are they able to recall specific words, numbers and phrases?
Do they appear attentive, distracted or able to concentrate?
Are they able to think in an abstract manner?

Orientation and Sensorium example
David's level of consciousness appears alert and he appears orientated to time, place and person. David reports that it is Sunday 5th July 2015, he is aware that he is being interviewed at The Smith Memorial Hospital in Melbourne and can remember the assessor's name. David is able to count backwards in 7's from 100 to 51, recall 3 words after 5 minutes and recall a phrase during the assessment. David appears to possess an appropriate level of current news events and he appears attentive and able to concentrate on the assessment process. David is able to recall a childhood memory, when he was at the beach with his family and also an event that he participated in yesterday. Both David's short-term and long-term memory appears intact, although these were not formally assessed.

Chapter 13: Insight and Judgement

Insight and judgement are key elements of the MSE, most particularly relating to making decisions about safety and risk.

Both insight and judgement can be described as absent, partial or limited, and full.

Insight relates to an individual's:

- Acknowledgement that they may be experiencing a mental illness.
- Understanding of possible treatment options and adherence.
- Ability to identify signs and symptoms of their potential mental illness.

Judgement relates to an individual's:

- Problem-solving ability and decision-making processes.
- Understanding of the consequences of their actions.

Prompt questions

What level of insight do they possess?
What level of judgement do they possess?
Can you provide evidence to support their level of insight and judgement?

Insight and Judgement example

David's level of insight into his current circumstances appears full, as evidenced by his ability to acknowledge his current grief and loss, treatment options and ability to identify early warning signs. David's level of judgement appears full, as evidenced by his ability to problem solve, make informed decisions and understand the consequences of his actions.

Chapter 14: Putting it all together

David Smith is a 42-year old Australian male. David reports that he is 185 cm tall and weighs 90 kilograms, and he appears to be of normal build. David appears younger than his stated age and he is wearing clean clothing that consists of a short-sleeved t-shirt, shorts, running shoes, a baseball cap and sunglasses, which are appropriate for the weather, as it is warm and sunny at the time of the assessment. David's hygiene appears intact and he has short clean and well-groomed hair and there is no evidence of body odour. David reports that he had a shower prior to the assessment.

David's facial expression appears sad, as evidenced by his continued tearfulness and he reports that his dog passed away today. David appears kind and interactive, as he is able to engage in conversation appropriately with obvious eye contact throughout the assessment. David does not appear uncoordinated and his rate of movement appears normal. David appears to actively engage in the assessment and he does not display any agitation, confrontation or dissatisfaction. David states *"thank you for listening to me"*.

David's speech appears to be of normal rate, flow and volume. David does not appear to raise his voice during the course of the interview. He appears coherent and his responses appear relevant to the conversation. David displays normal responsiveness to the assessor questions and he appears to offer normal quantity of information.

David describes his mood, as *"I'm not feeling too happy at the moment as my dog passed away today and I feel really sad"*. David's affect appears flat, which is appropriate to the situation he describes. David appears tearful throughout the interview. David's mood and affect appear congruent.

David's thought form appears logical and relevant to the conversation. David responds to each question logically and does not appear to offer illogical responses. For example, David was asked, *"Tell me more about your dog"*. David's response was *"my dog was a Border collie and his name was Duke. I know that he passed away today and I miss him terribly"*. David's response appears relevant to the subject matter. David does not appear to display any abnormal form of thought.

David does not appear to be experiencing, nor does he admit to, any current delusions, over-valued ideas, obsessions, phobias, preoccupations and harmful thoughts towards himself or others. David does not express any risk concerns relating to his own health or the health of others.

David expresses his current preoccupation with the death of his dog, however it is not clinically significant and it is in context with his current experience of grief and loss. David states that, "*if I need extra support regarding the death of Duke I will get it, but my family and friends have said that they will support me to organize a funeral and celebration for my dog in the next few days*".

David does not appear to be experiencing any current perceptual disturbance, as evidenced by his current denial of suffering from hallucinations, delusions or illusions. David denies any history of experiencing perceptual disturbance.

David's level of consciousness appears alert and he appears orientated to time, place and person. David reports that it is Sunday 5th July 2015, he is aware that he is being interviewed at The Smith Memorial Hospital in Melbourne and can remember the assessor's name. David is able to count backwards in 7's from 100 to 51, recall 3 words after 5 minutes and recall a phrase during the assessment.

David appears to possess an appropriate level of current news events and he appears attentive and able to concentrate on the assessment process. David is able to recall a childhood memory, when he was at the beach with his family and also an event that he participated in yesterday. Both David's short-term and long-term memory appears intact, although these were not formally assessed.

David's level of insight into his current circumstances appears full, as evidenced by his ability to acknowledge his current grief and loss, treatment options and ability to identify early warning signs. David's level of judgement appears full, as evidenced by his ability to problem solve, make informed decisions and understand the consequences of his actions.

Conclusion

In conclusion, it is imperative that the assessor conducts a thorough and systematic assessment. If the assessor builds a therapeutic relationship based on trust, empathy, unconditional positive regard, active listening and therapeutic engagement, the individual being assessed is more likely to engage in the assessment process and appropriate health outcomes can be achieved.

References

1. Lakeman, R. (1995). *The mental status examination*. Testandcalc.com, Australia.

2. Patrick, J. (2000). *Mental status examination rapid record form*. Melbourne, Australia.

3. Ensor, R. (2005). *Mental state examination*. Division of Cevado Technologies, U.S.A.

4. Kiran, C., & Chaudhury, S. (2009). Understanding delusions. *Industrial Psychiatry Journal, 18*(1), 3-18.

5. MH4OT. (2016). *MH4OT glossary*. Australia.

6. Merriam-Webster.com. (2016). *Pseudohallucination*. Merriam-Webster: U.S.A.

Printed in Great Britain
by Amazon